© September, 2007 Warhorse Publication

ISBN NO. 0-9755272-1-5

All rights are reserved by the Warhorse Publications. No part of this book may be reproduced, copies or utilized in any form or by any means, electronic or mechanical, photocopying, recording or any other means that can reproduce the contents and information in this book, without the written permission from the copyright holder, prior to the using any of the information in this book.

Warhorse Publications
P.O. Box 280724
Nashville, Tennessee 37207

Price $11.50 Retail

Contents

Introduction

Understanding the Source

To get a complete understanding about the material in this book, I am led to give the readers the opportunity to reach a conclusion for themselves and determine whether the issues discussed herein are mere coincidences or acts of divine intervention. My views are based on information provided to me by my mother in conjunction with actual events I have experienced and are discussed herein.

At an early age my mother informed me that I was born with a veil over my face. Not knowing exactly what that meant, she explained to me that I am able to see things that other people cannot see. The revelations that I get are not in the form of a vision. It seems as though the answer comes immediately to my thoughts when the problem or need is heard. This is not a process that happens at every occasion. As close as I can understand it seems as though the revelation manifest itself when there is a conflict involving the needs of a righteous or good hearted person and a conflict with good and bad. This is not a process that I can call upon at any time for any person. It does not work like that. This is not a process that I can call upon to prove a point that these revelations appear to me.

When I began to receive these revelations, I did not know how to communicate the intended purpose without offending the person it was directed to and to give an example: I was in graduate school at Tennessee State University School of Education. On one occasion while in the classroom with approximately thirty (30) other students, I received a revelation. Most of the students were teachers in various school districts. One of the students, Mia J. is a guidance counselor with the public system in Nashville, Tennessee was having a conversation with another student, Dr. Johnetta M., who was an employee with the Campus Security Department. I overheard the conversation when Mia informed her of her intended future wedding. I immediately responded without any consideration and said, "You should reconsider because it is not going to workout.". . . and she replied, "You don't even know me or my fiancée who in the hell do you think you are to through salt on my wedding?" and it got the attention of the entire class. The revelation was not showing any fault on her part, but her intended husband was not being honest with her and not worthy of her as a partner. The marriage lasted for a short time and we are friends to this date. She has a new friend in her life and she is happy to this day.

The same incident happened again with a different student in the classroom at Middle Tennessee State University. The exact same revelation manifested itself before a full classroom of teachers. There was a difference in this revelation. This marriage could not work because the young lady could not be in love with anyone except herself and she wanted to get married for revenge against someone who would not marry her. I never knew her name.

Many individuals attempt to make rules and procedures for God to perform his promise of giving blessings. There are individuals that proclaim that God has preordained methods that he follows to give blessings. There is nothing in the Bible to support that illusion. Many so called religious Christians advocate and tell their collogues that 'gambling' is a sin, but the word 'gamble' is not located in the Bible anywhere. However it does mention 'games of chance', but 'games of chance' is basically what the American culture is all about. An example for blessings on gambling is when I was in the Sam's Clothing Store on 5th.Avenue in Nashville, Tennessee. I was buying several summer casual suits. The saleslady, Doris T. said to me, " You are buying a lot of clothes today." and I said that God has blessed me to be able to buy them. She replied, " I sure wish God will bless me, I am trying to by a house." and I was instructed to tell her to play 683 in the Illinois lottery with the street bookies. She said that she needed all the money she had to put down on her house. I was further instructed to give her $100.00 and I told her to put it all on 683 that evening. That evening 683 fell straight. I went back to buy more clothes the next day, when I asked her if she played the number and she hesitated and said yes. Because she was slow answering, I asked if she played the whole $100.00 and she said no, she played $1.00 and I could see the hurt in her eyes. If she had followed the instructions she would have won $70,000.00 to pay cash for her house. Being disobedient, she only won $700.00.

When you buy stock and bonds, you are involved in a 'game of chance'. You are literally putting up your money and hoping to gain a profit from your investment.

6.

This is also gambling. When you show up on a job to get a weekly salary, you are gambling that the business will not go bankrupt before giving you a paycheck. In the next example, the young lady did not perform any gambling activities. I was the person that received a substantial blessing, with instructions to count out a specific portion, which I did and placed a rubber band around to keep it together. I was instructed to drive from my home down Clarksville Highway, in Nashville, a few blocks from my home. I was led to drive into the Sonic Drive In, to the last car going in. I had no prior knowledge of who would be there, but upon arriving, I recognized the driver to be Vickie, H., the Supervisor of the Records Department at Tennessee State University. I was led to go to the passenger side and give the money to

7.

the passenger in the front seat, who was Lisa, G. and I did that. Upon leaving, I heard Vickie tell her to throw the money out, but I kept walking back to my car. Approximately two days later Lisa called me and thanked me. She explained by saying, "I don't know how you knew that I needed the money. My husband was injured and not able to work and I went to the altar Sunday and prayed for the exact amount of money that you gave me. I will pay you back when I can." , and I responded immediately and told her that I did not give her anything that required repayment. I was just the messenger and there is nothing to be repaid.

I will give a final example to show that God protects his believers at all times and take on your battles for you. God used me to remove some of the most powerful men in America from their powerful positions for simply abusing their powers and not performing their duties they had sworn to do. One thing that you must remember at all times, God is alive and he holds you to any oath that you may take in his name. You may not believe it but words have power and without even knowing it you can condemn yourself to hell without ever knowing it. When you take on the position to abuse your lawful powers to do unjust dealings, you will pay the ultimate price. The first will be at the cost of the closest love of your life. It may be a person, property or position.

The example I promised is based on the fact I was wrongfully criminally prosecuted in Tennessee Criminal Court without an indictment to support the criminal charge. The Court of Criminal Appeals reversed the conviction but Joe Henry, Tennessee Supreme Court Justice wrote the opinion that reinstated the conviction. He was the picture of good health and jogged five miles (5) everyday before getting on the bench. Shortly thereafter he had a heart attack and died and every justice in the Tennessee Supreme Court that concurred with him is off the bench or/and dead. Every justice in the U.S. Supreme Court that refused to hear my case is off the bench except Justice Stevens who had been recently appointed to the court and had very little to do with my case. Every judge that has ever locked me up is off the bench. The trial judge in my case did not want to send me to prison, I wrote the Order of commitment and he signed it. His only wrong was to mock me in open court in front of several lawyers and people waiting to have their case heard. He also has an illness that he can overcome, if he can set aside his pride to do what is necessary. A federal judge, called me a 'habitual liar' in a court case that I was not involved in and he has a sickness he can't overcome because his pride won't allow him to do what is necessary. His statements was based on a report filed by Bill Mulkins, an F.B.I. Agent who is now deceased from a sickness that he could not overcome. His partner, Larry Olsen never disrespected me in any way at any time and he has lived a long and prosperous life and his seed will always be blessed. I had nothing to do with any of these events. God has defended me all of my life, in every incident.

I have only prayed for the recovery from illness for two individuals in my life. Dr. Paul Madden, a former instructor at Tennessee State University who was in a comma for several days. My prayers were motivated by his actions as a teacher that demonstrated a genuine concern for his students. He recovered and was a member of my dissertation committee at Tennessee State University. The other was former Tennessee Supreme Court Justice. My prayers were motivated based on the respect I developed from knowing him over thirty (30) years. My respect was based on the fact he knew what he wanted to accomplish and he stuck with his plan to accomplish his goal. I was never concerned about whether he liked me or not. I learned to respect him for being focused on his goal to succeed and stuck with his plan to accomplish his success. He has recovered and plays golf on a regular basis while this book is being written. When my case came before the Supreme Court he always recused himself. I have a love and respect for him as I would have for an older brother. By observing his success I gained respect for him doing what was necessary for him to accomplish his dreams in spite of all opposition. I learned to persevere and not allow petty distractions to cause me to take my eye off the ultimate prize to complete my dreams. Even though our beliefs were different it is the process of completion that matters.

The facts as stated in this introduction may be co-incidents or divine intervention and you being the reader can reach your own conclusion. I do not proclaim to be the God fearing person that I should be, but I am trying.

Chapter 1

Understanding the Power of the Anointed

Many of us read the Bible and do not understand exactly what is being said. I have a great respect for men that say God has chosen them to perform the religious duties that are assigned to those who are chosen. Even though the Bible warns us to be aware of false prophets, no one is qualified to pick and choose who was not actually called by God to conduct these duties. I have to accept the position that all people are not on the same cultural and educational level and the selection of prophets was probably selected based on different cultural and educational levels to complete the communication process in our churches. It must be considered and understood that God said if he called you, he would prepare you. He never said that he would prepare them overnight with all the information that is needed. In fact, there is no single individual that serves as a man of God that knows everything there is to know about the Bible, or the word of God. It must be understood that the learning process must come from one prophet to another to make the circle complete. Each individual have a different level of understanding and the teaching process must be performed by men traveling under the guides of ordained ministers as required in the American culture.

Since we are also warned in advance to be aware of false prophets. No one has to point them out. They will point themselves out by their words that contradict the spirit of the Bible. The excuses used by many followers is, the issue of being a false prophet is between the preacher and God. That is also true, but once God has revealed the truth to you and you choose to follow a false prophet 'free will' makes you accountable for your own actions. You may choose to follow them because they have a smooth voice to sing with and hold your attention during church services. You must remember that these are also qualities that the adversary possesses. In fact, Lucifer was the greatest singer in heaven before being expelled. Because many congregations consists of a large number of members does not mean that church is sanctioned under God. Free will gives you the ability to determine for yourself and it is then when you are accountable for your own actions.

Do not misunderstand what has been said so far. It is not every church that has a large congregation of members, led by false prophets either. It is not every minister that makes a mistake in the Sunday sermons that are not supported by the Bible considered as a false prophet. It is the intent that lies in his heart that will manifest itself to you and you that have ears will hear and those who have eyes will see. We must understand that our ministers are not perfect and we are not either. All of us make mistakes and errors on a regular basis. We must use our 'free will' to examine and consider the essence of the material that is being taught for continuity with the word as we read our Bible. Even though we listen to our ministers we have the obligation and responsibility to use our 'free will' to examine these statements for truth.

17.

Many individuals believe that even though they have reasonable knowledge of adultery and other sinful activities by their minister, they cannot be held accountable for his actions. Bear in mind, any person that consistently act contrary to what is written in the Ten Commandments are considered to be unclean in the eyes of GOD and you have been instructed to 'get out from among them'. There are ministers that tell their congregation, "don't do as I do, but do as I say do." . . . as if this justified them being qualified to perform their appointed duties of the Church. Contrary to whatever your beliefs may be, you will also be held accountable for your actions if you knowingly and willingly continues to stay within their presence and the same sinful conduct is constantly going on. This principle has overflowed into the concept of enforcement of the civilized laws of society. If you witness a person being murdered and you failed or refused to do anything or call the local law enforcement authorities in many jurisdictions will prosecute you as an accessory for not doing anything. Whether an individual qualifies to be a 'false prophet' is not within my powers to judge and no one else, unless they have a heaven or hell to elevate or condemn the prophet to. Certainly, there is no human being on earth that has such powers. However, your eyes and ears are the only sources that God has granted you to make decisions for yourself and a reason to exercise 'free will' to make your choices to stay where you are, or to get out from among the situation you are under. There are several incidents that I have witnessed, but I do not attempt to label these individuals as 'false prophets'. Two Individual's that I have the greatest respect for made statements on national television that I have a problem understanding, which are:

The Bible tells us that, "It is easier for a camel to go through the eye of a needle, than for a rich man to enter into the kingdom of God." Bishop T.D. Jakes said that statement was made in reference to a path that a camel travels, but I have found nothing in the Bible to support that position. I believed that if there was a path involved, there is only one such path and the Bible would have read as, 'the needle' rather than 'a needle'. However, I also know that there is another meaning to that phrase and only those who have ears can hear it and those who have eyes can see the true meaning. If there was no other meaning involved it would be clear that God has the imperfection to error, which is not likely because God has made many man rich beyond their wildest dreams. Certainly he would not deliberately condemn any man by banning his chances from entering the kingdom because of his riches. First we must understand what God has defined as a rich man, which by no means has any relations to his acquired success with money and worldly goods. God has said that the love of money is the root of all evil. A rich man is considered to be a person that has considerable wealth and riches and have so greater love for his money that he is selfish and refuses to help those who are unfortunate and unable to help themselves. God blesses people through other people. When you are so selfish that you refuse to help

21.

those in need, you take the risk of banning yourself from entering the kingdom of God. When you help friends and family you are still functioning within the rims of selfishness. When you help a stranger and a beggar that is in need, this is when you rise to the level of being unselfish. It is not necessary to give money when money will add to the 'beggar'' problems, especially when it is obvious they have an addiction problem. Offer to buy food or clothing or to pay a bill. The Bible tells us, if a beggar asks for your coat, give it to him. It did not say give him a sleeve or collar to the coat.

The Bible tells us to 'Judge not that ye be not judged.' and on one occasion I witnessed Rev. Jimmy Swaggart making a public confession for his past act of indiscretion. On another occasion I witnessed him mentioning, Bill Gates of the Micro Soft Corporation. He admitted that he did not know if Mr. Gates was saved, but he added, "I doubt it.". Since he has no heaven or hell to send Mr. Gates to, he lacks any authority to judge since there is a bigger question mark before his own name of being saved. Just because you profess to the world that you are saved don't mean that you are actually saved. Man has always been able to make his mouth say whatever he wants to hear. This is commonly know as an untrue statement.

Many churches will give a collar or a sleeve when it is within their power to give the coat. Disobedience has always been the downfall of man. Out of selfishness, Churches have a tendency to exercise a great margin of selfishness, especially among strangers who are not part of their congregation. All Churches are locked so tight that Jesus can't get inside to pray. If Churches were truly Houses of God, there would be no locks on the doors and there would be a keeper of the house. It is written that God made man in his own image, but man has placed limitations of his ability to love. The supreme duty that God has placed on man, was the single instruction that Jesus asked of his twelve Apostles, "to love one another as I have loved you.", but no one has ever learned to follow that one single instruction to this date, because of selfishness and self preservation at some level. Man has applied one obligation towards his family and a different standard toward God's family. Man has allows his seed to return home at any time rather than to be homeless. If the Churches were truly a house of God, then God's seed

24.

would be allowed to enter the Church at anytime to rest and for shelter when his children are homeless. Man has a greater fear that thieves will steal from the Church, but if the Church really belong to God, that is a single issue for God and man has never been appointed to conduct the affairs of God. Man has appointed himself to make specific conduct that is not defined in the Bible as a sin when he is not capable of attending his own affairs. That is exactly what caused Lucifer to become Satin. You cannot be the Master and the Servant. The lesson given to Satin should be obvious to the believers of Christianity. The problem is man is still performing the first trick created by man. The very first trick created by man was to make his mouth say whatever he wants to hear and not realizing his words contradict those in the Bible.

There is nothing in the Bible that restricts God to a specific and set way to give blessings. Man does not have the ability to select the means or the methods God will use to grant blessings. Since man have the gift of 'free will', then certainly God has 'free will' also to do as he pleases. There must be a clear understanding that there are no restrictions on God and there have never been restrictions on how God will answer prayers. Likewise it must be understood that man lacks the ability to place restrictions on God. In fact, man is incapable of controlling his own actions through restrictions. I have heard individuals who travel under the cloak of religion as ministers say publicly, there were some issues in the Bible that are irrelevant. However, if the Bible was truly written by men who were inspired by God, if one single

26.

issue or statement is irrelevant, then the whole book is irrelevant. That individual failed to meet the requirements to hear and see the truth and that single statement placed him on the rim of a true false prophet. It is a prophet's duty to defend the Bible and it's entire contents. It is Satin's desire to attack the Bible and create doubt about its meaning among the believers. A true Christian will not avoid explaining the contents of the Bible for fear of insulting a culture or placing one culture's belief over another. We did not write a single statement in the Bible and we don't have the authority or right to refuse to answer, when there is a question involving the truth and we have the knowledge to do so. I use the term 'we' with respect to individuals that have ears to hear and eyes to see with an understanding heart.

There will be times when one individual will have a completely different understanding of what the scriptures have said. There are many occasions when one part of the Bible will warn you of a sin and at another part, permission is given to do the exact same act, without the label of a sin. One example is in the contents of the Ten Commandments we have been instructed not to kill by the language which say's, "Thou shall not kill". At another section of the Bible it gives permission to kill by the language which say's, "To every thing there is a season, and a time to every purpose under the heaven: ' A time to kill, and a time to heal;'. . . and this is the type of statements that require the reader to have ears and eyes for understanding. The casual reader believes the first as stated in the Ten Commandments relates only to humans.

To the contrary, it plainly forbids a deliberately killing of any form of life without a reason or purpose. The latter is self-explanatory because we understand the necessity to kill as a requirement since man is at the top of the food chain. The necessity to kill is accepted to maintain order in our society.

The basic cultural conflicts are caused because there is a lack of knowledge and understanding in the culture's true history. One culture have a history that survived on hiding the truth from their own seed hoping that the truth will be lost forever. It must be understood that the truth can never be lost. God chose individuals to reveal the truth to, so it can never be lost. Events that occurred more than a thousand years or since the beginning of time can be revealed to the chosen few at any time God desire to do so. One culture has a past that is based on shame that is considered to be horrible by the standards as set out by the American standards. The very thing that one culture is ashamed of is the very thing another culture is proud of, simply because the latter have no concept of exactly what the truth is. That is by strategic design because of the foolish concept on superior behavior first imposed upon them. This method angered God because no culture is superior over another. At this point, the true history is not important. It is relevant but not important enough to interfere with the anointed performing their duties to teach believers to love one another as God has loved us and without hesitation and reservation.

30.

The anointed has the duty to teach believers that "African American" does not mean you are Black. It means that your ancestors came from Africa but you live in America today. According to Genesis, everyone in America is 'African American'. In fact, if the Garden of Eden was located on the African continent as stated in Genesis, individuals in Japan would be African Japanese, those in China would be African Chinese. The same logic would apply to all other countries, if Adam and Eve were the parents of all humans.

It must be taught that Black and White are not races. Human is a race. Black and White are colors and cultures.

Chapter 2

Words have Power

A prudent person should take the time to chose words to communicate with. Believe it or not, words are powerful and can serve a two-fold purpose as a double edge sword. Even words that are expressed in humor or play during a daily conversation can have a dramatic effect on a person as well as you. A negative word to a person can result in negative actions against that person even though its effect cannot be seen. The mind receives the negative word and it is planted in the mind as a seed in the earth and will grow as a plant. Especially when raising children care in the selection of words in the presence of young and impressionable ears is necessary. The words used to criticize or communicate with children are like loading a computer database to store information for future purposes. As long as that child live those words will be remembered until senility sets in. If negative words were used to describe that child, most likely there will be no visible signs of ambition to suggest that child will have a desire to reach its peak potential level of intelligence. However, there are exceptions to that opinion. A strong willed individual will develop a desire to succeed in spite of all opposition. This is the attitude that was present in some of the Negro slaves that saw members of the Caucasian culture reading. Even thou reading was forbidden by slave owners, the older slaves accepted that tradition and tried to impress that idea upon the younger slaves. Some of the youngsters accepted that tradition but as with everything else, there were exceptions to the rule and some of them wanted to learn to read. If there was to be success in learning to read, it had to be a secret and they dared not tell anyone. This secret could not be shared with anyone not even to another slave.

Communication with words has a powerful affect in every situation in the world today. Using the right words at the right time can express many emotions such as anger, love, hate, intentions, desires and any other emotion that is possible. Words used out of anger can have a lasting effect on any person, even though it appears the words were ignored. Long after the conversation when the words were planted in the memory bank of your mind, you will have flashes about the words that were used. You will think of words you should have said and things you should have done. When this happens the seed words are growing. This is when you must use self-discipline to restrain your actions. There have been situations when individuals allow words to grow to the extent they are motivated to return to confront the person again and in many situations results in a violent confrontation. That is why judges are prone to impose a more harsh and sever punishment. You had the time to cool off and this is referred to a 'cooling off period'. When your anger exceeds the 'cooling off period' the words have grown as a young child grows. Words grow from idle words of anger to a different stage called 'intent'. Intent is the stage of growth that convinces a person that there is a need to do something else to get satisfaction for the words that were used on them. This is the kind of mentality that animals rely on for survival. Only humans have the mentality to read this book and being so, humans have a sense that lower forms of animals do not have. We have the ability to reason and exercise 'free will' that animals do not have. We have the ability to walk away and ask God to take on our battle for us and to take that issue from your mind. The problem is most people allow pride to interfere in their lives. Pride is the vanity of a foolish person. The word 'Intent' is the mother of all crimes and before a crime can be committed, 'intent' must be present.

The word 'rejection' is also a powerful word that many people do not like and refuse to accept. When you refuse to accept the consequences of 'rejection', you are inviting the word 'intent' to come into your life. It is obvious that when 'intent' comes into your life you are about to do something that will interrupt the normal flow of at least two lives. Yours and some other individual that may have demonstrated some form of 'rejection' to you. Even though you have an investment in a relationship either business or personal there is always the option of walking away as though it is a bad investment in stock. You can always get more opportunities to make other investments as long as you are able to exercise 'free will', but when you place additional limitations on yourself, you lose.

That is why it is important for a married couple not to retire for the night in an angry mood. One half of the couple may not wake up and the other half will probably go though the remaining portion of life with the regret of not saying simple words of apology. It is not important who is wrong. Depending on the words that were said, an apology could be very hard to accept. That is why a person should be ready to accept the consequences for choosing the wrong words. There are words when used inappropriately even God will not forgive. If man was made in God's image, how can you expect another human to forgive you when you use the words that are strictly a 'no no term' that must never be used under any circumstance. In the initial stages of a relationship many couples set ground rules. These rules are considered to be boundaries that cannot be crossed at any time, for any reason. The only solution for breaking these rules is to part company. One partner may say they forgive the other but they cannot forget what has happened. That statement clearly means that they are incapable of forgiving and the only solution is to get away from each other on a permanent basis.

Some of the greatest men of our time have experienced the power of words. Most of them never thought about the incidents that initiated the results. The world witnessed an incident when President Clinton used the military forces to compel the leaders of Haiti to leave the country. One of the officials told President Clinton that he would send a mass of spirits upon him to revenge his cause. I do not remember the exact words that were used, but the world knows of the consequence of those words. Soon thereafter every possible means of embarrassment a man can endure fell upon the President and he was marked in the pages of history as no other President has been since the beginning of American politics. When these words were spoken it was amusing to the world and most Americans though this type of talk or verbal expression was comical or amusing and made mockery at that individual.

When you use words to cause discomfort to others, for an unjust cause, that fate will return to you. Never cause more pains to happen to others through words, than you can stand to bear when they return to you. Paraphrasing a statement in the Bible, "He that diggeth a ditch shall fall therein", but the scriptures says, "He made a pit, and digged it, and is fallen into the ditch which he made" [Psalm 7:15]. As I interpret that statement, I believe that when you seek to cause harm to others, you will suffer the consequences for your labor to plot against another person.

During your daily travels while in your car or walking, use words to ask for the desires of your heart. Speak the words that will bring comfort and relief to you. It is written in the Bible that instructs you to ask and it shall be given. It said nothing about thinking about it and it shall be given. Pick and choose the surroundings and environment to ask for your desires. You do not need an audience. Even when you conduct the prayer in Church, it should not be done to impress the congregation. Long drawn out speeches on the knees is nothing short of vanity. If we are more responsive to short and straight to the point conversations, then it must be the same with God since we are made in his image. When your heart is clean and your intentions are sincere, use short, plain and simple words to ask for what you want. It does not matter whether you are asking God or a person. Remember God give blessings through other people. Even people that you believe will not help you, God will touch their heart and they will not be able to refuse you. The right words to any person will grant your desires when it is within their powers to do so and they have the means to help you. God has placed earthly angles for all of his believers and you will not know who yours are until you ask for help. Many of these individuals do not know that they are assigned to conduct divine business and do not know they have no control in these matters. Often when it is done and at a later time, even they will question themselves on why they provided assistance to someone they never had a reason to do for in the past. This is when your blessings come back to you as a reward. Joel Osteen said give freely with the expectation of receiving a blessing. I tested that theory. My job pays me with direct deposit, which hits the ATM at 12:01 am on Friday morning. I arrived at the Exxon Service Station on the corner of 12th. Avenue and Broad Street at the above time when a young Black man was standing near the door asking for money. He asked all of the Caucasian customers, but he never asked me. No one gave him anything while I watched. I checked my balance and withdrew $20.00 from my account and gave it to the beggar. When I got to my car I spoke the words, "I gave my money with the expectation of getting a blessing.". . .the next day I received an unexpected gift of $175.00. This reinforced my belief that words do have power.

43.

Chapter 3

God is an Observer

Things that we see on a daily basis, we take for granted that no one really cares. Bear in mind regardless of how small or petty we believe an issue to be God is aware of the smallest act of injustice and wrongful deeds that are inflicted on his children. He will give power to those who seek it, knowing that they will use it to destroy themselves through 'free will' and then punish them.

Even though I have never talked with an American Indian about their affairs especially when it concerns the gambling casinos. God recognized the fact the distribution of wealth has never been distributed among the blood relations that are entitled to receive a share. He knows that the Mexican's that are crossing the boarders into the United States because of the poverty in Mexico are actually Native American related. Their ancestors were chased into Mexico during the days of the civil war with the Indians. They are simply trying to come home. They learned to speak Spanish from the explorers that settled in Mexico. God will impress upon the U.S. Government for Indian Affairs and the Internal Revenue to create a DNA database with tribes that are receiving a share of the gambling funds, to be compared with Mexicans that volunteer to be compared with the established tribes. He knows that the tribes will refuse and oppose the creation of the DNA database based on greed. Those who refuse will be subjected to elimination of their Native American status and subjected to income taxes as other American citizens, until they can proved they are Native Americans through the DNA database.

God is also aware of the fact Mexico cannot defend itself and depends upon the protection of the United States, if it is confronted with a situation too large or great to defend against. Eventually God will touch the hearts of politicians of the two Countries to include Mexico as a State within the boundaries of the United States to decrease the poverty level in Mexico. The President of Mexico will become the Governor. This is done most likely with a buyout too great for interested parties to refuse. Major corporations will move to Mexico in the interest of profits and savings they can get, due to the low wage standards. Those that act fast will benefit, but eventually wages will rise on a competitive level with other corporations in Texas. That is the only solution to illegal boarder crossing into the United States.

That will stop fugitives from fleeing from the United States into Mexico to avoid criminal prosecutions. The U. S. Government will build the majority of federal prisons in Mexico and in areas that are within the deserts, away from civilian populations. Prison escapes will be impossible and can only be successful with the help of prison officials. The only boarder the United States will have to deal with is the Canadian boarder. Only chances to enter will be through local docks where ships enter and private boats travel through the oceans and seas.

There will be a mass examination of containers entering the United States and less concern with those leaving the United States. More concern will be directed towards transportation on all roads and highways.

Even incidents that occurred long ago, God is aware and he will remove individuals that have cold hearts from their positions of power until he permit the quality of person of his choice to do the right thing. That person will have the qualities and abilities to perform the required duties with compassion, sympathy, justice and mercy. They will have to exercise their power toward others in the exact same process, as they would like to be treated, if they were in the same situation. God has recognized the fact that men when elevated to power over other people, tends to forget their limitations and act as though they are entitled to be a Supreme Being as the Master. Man is designed to be the servant of God, who is the Master. Man cannot be the Master and the Servant and a prudent individual with power should remember that. God is aware of the fact man is constantly seeking ways to exclude him from his own creation. The U. S. Supreme Court has said that there must be a separation between Church and State. God is aware of that and he has responded, but through arrogance men of average intelligence have not noticed. There is not one single judge in power and on the bench in the U.S. Supreme Court that set the precedent to exclude God from business dealing with State Government. In reality, there can be no separation between State and Church because State issues are also Church issues. All State laws are derivatives from the Ten Commandments. Marriage was first a Church issue but States began selling marriage license. Murder was first prohibited in the Ten Commandments but States prosecutes for killing.

In essence there is no possible way there can be a separation between Church and State. This Country was built and established on religious principles and doctrines. That is exactly why the Pilgrims came here in search for land that would allow them to exercise their rights to worship as they please. The desired right at that time was Christianity. This country gives respect through the United States Constitution to other religions that may come to the United States. To allow non-citizens or immigrants to change or dictate the rules this country was built on defies the efforts our ancestors fought for and died to protect. If I am allowed to move into your house, I must respect the rules of the house. Certainly your house rules will let me practice my own religion, but you will not allow my religion to change your house rules.

50.

It is these religious house rules that allowed the head of house to set the standards for civil behavior for their children and introduced religious character on respect for others. Our Constitution was never designed or meant to allow individual rights to be tampered with, based on other cultures and their religion. The American traditions survived for hundreds of years without a serious flaw until its process was allowed to diminish, which caused our children to stray. Our children developed less respect for other's rights, which was a starting point. They even have very little respect for family members and do harm to each other on a regular basis. They have very little knowledge of God and Religion, which was introduced at an early age in the past in our schools. Religion is a part of history and the Bible is the oldest history book known to the American culture. The Bible becomes a 'Holy Book' when the reader start practicing the methods of praying. If the schools are designed for teaching our children, they must be allowed to learn every phase of life skills that are necessary for survival in a civilized society. Our own Supreme Court has said that the citizens of this country must have 'NOTICE' of any and all conduct that is allowed and that which is prohibited. When you exclude religious teachings of all kind from public schools, the states have failed to provide 'NOTICE' of the conduct that is acceptable in a civilized society. Conduct that is influenced by religious beliefs to love and respect each other. Our laws are willing to freely execute our children for not having 'NOTICE' to respect the lives of others. The parents of our children

52.

grew up under these conditions and do not allow teachers to use their skills to teach that child right from wrong. That parent, not being aware is setting that child up for failure. The police department will inherit the neglected duty to punish that child through beatings on the streets, and probably result in a killing by police. Parents being over concerned that discipline will not be distributed equally, will subject their child to unequal punishment. There is no valid argument to that position. In fact, teachers should be required to subject unequal punishment to show our children at an early age that they will be subjected to unfair treatment in life at some point. This will build strength and character in the child and teach them methods to make complaints, rather than shoot a child, or adult because of their terms of 'disrespect'. It is obvious that the methods being used must be changed. Our children are committing crimes in the courtrooms and in front of judges. They are killing their own parents on a regular basis. They are taking human life for sport and initiation in street gangs, without remorse. Human lives are being wasted simply because one party cannot accept rejection and commits murder suicides and taking their children with them. Parents ask God why he allows their children to be killed in our schools, but forgot they asked God to stay out of the schools and off the school property. Even God is required to look at the killings from across the streets and not allowed to interfere, because of man exercising his God given right to 'free will'.

Federal and State politicians are sworn into public offices on the Bible. The politician's argument rests on the assumption that Americans have the right to worship, as they please, but not on State property. It is clear that there is no valid argument. It is the people that make up a State and it is the people that make up the Church. Even the Government is the people also and it is impossible to separate people from people without violating federal laws prohibiting discrimination. The separation of people for any reason is segregation and is prohibited by federal law under Title 42, §1983 of the U.S. Codes. Man has always tried to pick and choose specific occasions they want to include God in their lives. We pray and ask God to protect our children serving in the military but we want him to stay away from our children when they are in schools. As a result God is not allowed to protect our children from harm because we exercised 'free will' to keep him away. We don't want school teachers to discipline our children to teach them right from wrong, but we allow policemen to beat them later on and it is alright if the policemen kill them because we failed as parents to raise them in accord with the word. We have been instructed in the Bible of the consequences of not properly disciplining our children. It clearly says, "Spare the rod and spoil the child". As a result of such failures the Criminal Justice System is a booming business. Children are conducting crimes on a daily basis that adults were committing in the past. This is the consequence of disobedience of the word through the exercise of 'free will'. Parents use whatever words is convenient at the time to talk to their children when angry. It is these words that plant the seed to determine the future personality of that child. Whatever words you use on a child at the age of five will be remembered throughout the life of that child until senility sets in at old age. If you tell the child at an early age he or she is nothing and will never be nothing they will believe that and less efforts will be applied to dispute that belief. Children have young and impressionable ears and whatever you say to them are the words that are actively molding that child to be whatever they will be. If your words created a criminal then don't blame the child, put the blame where it belongs, on yourself. If a child is programmed to believe that he is nothing, then it will have no foundation to build anything on. Every creation

57.

that is made has a foundation and for a child to be a success, there has to be a foundation to support success. If that child becomes a criminal, that too has to have a foundation. Whatever words you use around that child at the impressionable years start the building of the foundation for the survival of that child. Some parents believe that the right to discipline their child will promote bias and prejudice in the execution of discipline through corporal punishment. Even if that is the case, teachers will not kill or inflict cruel and unusual punishment that amounts to child abuse. The introduction to bias and prejudice at an early age will introduce that child to the realities of the world that life is not fair on any level. They can be prepared to handle such situations when they reach maturity. They can learn how to make complaints

58.

and that is important for the growth of a child. It teaches a child that even the authority figures can be wrong and they should be able to have the knowledge of making complaints against authority figures as teachers and enjoy the satisfaction of getting an apology or explanation for actions they believed to be unjust. This is the American way. Otherwise children react through violence on individuals for actions that may have occurred unintentional. This is what children call 'disrespect'. Adversity at an early age teaches our children to question the actions and intentions of others and by doing that, they would avoid senseless acts of violence and aggression. In most situations children displays the kind of aggression they are a custom to in their normal family environment. That is why it is necessary for teachers to have the opportunity to introduce a child to a setting that is accepted by our culture away from violence. When that child reject that view, the teacher must have the authority to set ground rules and on some occasions various forms or methods is required. For the survival of our children, the thought and concept that they are untouchable should be eliminated from that child's memory process by any means and as soon as possible. Mainly because that child will reach the conclusion, since the teacher cannot touch them they are untouchable. They fail to realize the fact the child sitting next to them may kill them if they cross the line with a fellow student. When children knows the limitation a teacher can act, they tend to react in a more aggressive manner towards authority. This is why a child's greatest enemy is the parent. The parent sets that

60.

child up for failure in society by depriving it of the opportunity to learn the skills for anger management. In some cultures anger is a normal expression that can only be resolved through violence. Unfortunately these cultures exist in the United States and clashes with the American way of life. It is these clashes that made the Criminal Justice System a big business in America. Our culture has created a child protection group under the various local governments that is against all forms of physical punishment on children and influence politicians to create laws prohibiting a parent from exercising the use of the rod as explained in the Bible. We as a civilized society must realize the fact that, power in the hands of a foolish person is like placing a weapon in the hands of a child. It will be constantly misused. Laws are created to compel the child to be placed on the path for being a statistic in the Criminal Justice System. If laws prevent the child from being taught right from wrong, then wrong is a path that is available for the exploring and the consequences leaves a criminal conviction. Laws allow such convictions to remain as a label to prevent that child from ever recovering from that wrong. That individual has his or her future set on a course which there is no return and is contrary to God's word. If God can forgive you for past sins of aggressions, who are you to hold another individual accountable for past criminal acts of aggression. Man has never learned to love one another as God has loved them or treat others, as they want to be treated in the same or similar situations.

Even incidents that appear to have little impact on the world as a whole, God is still watching and he will touch the hearts of those involved to rectify many of them. After all these years and the world have long since forgotten, God still remembers the wrong that was imposed upon Vanessa Williams, the first Black Miss America. He knows that there were many Caucasian winners that made more drastic mistakes than she did and was allowed to keep their crowns. His plan was to allow Ms. Williams to exercise her 'free will' to determine her destiny and prepare her for pains that were in her path. She endured those pains with a greater level of tenacity than she would have, had she not been introduced to pains and disappointments at an early age. It was her destiny to learn to trust her own judgment rather than to rely on individuals who she had trusted. God will touch the hearts of those in the position to reevaluate her cause during the Miss America contest and give her the proper recognition that she deserved because there was no iron clad definition to justify her crown being taken away. Even the U.S. Supreme Court has said in so many cases and on so many occasions, there must be clear and plain notice in writing as to exactly what kind of conduct that is prohibited and what is allowed. When this kind of 'Notice' is given everyone must comply with the conditions that are set out in writing. No one is immune or exempted from that standard, otherwise the process is contaminated and no one can be subjected to suffer for the consequences of their actions unless the same principle applies to all other constants. God will give them time to rectify their wrong and if they fail or refuse to do so, he will cause an interested party to come forth and reveal the exception to the world. If God can remove unjust men from the most powerful Court in the United States for arrogance and abuse of powers, certainly he can replace those in authority to do justice to Vanessa Williams and give her the Crown she earned and so much deserve. There is at least one Miss America with a shady past that will be revealed to the world when one interested party will expose that individual and the world know that Vanessa was treated with bias and prejudice and her crown will be reinstated to her.

God is even aware of the situation involving Pete Rose and the arrogance that is being imposed upon him. The reasons used to keep him from the Hall of Fame had nothing with his ability to play ball and he earned the right to be inducted into the Hall of Fame. What he was accused of is not an unusual act of conduct by ball players. Pete was not the first and certainly will not be the last to bet on his team to win. If he had placed a bet against his team and they lost there would be justification to inquire to determine if his conduct in the game was a determining factor in losing the game. Pete Rose will be inducted into the Hall of Fame and God is aware of the fact, removal of several individuals will be necessary to accomplish that deed. God only requires man to exercise 'free will' and to do his best in whatever task he takes on. There is no dispute that Mr. Rose earned the right to receive all of the recognition that is allowed to other players. The rules are contaminated when they can be interpreted and manipulated, rather than state specific conduct that is applied to all players. The investigation process should have included the manner the gambling act was engaged and the manner the act was discovered to bring charges against Mr. Rose. If there is the possibility of a conspiracy to prevent Mr. Rose from being inducted the investigative process should have documented that view. This is the main fault that God finds with man. They have a tendency to judge others in a manner that they do not want to be judged under similar and the same circumstances. The excuse that Mr. Rose denied betting for years should have no impact on his eligibility to qualify for the Hall of Fame. No one has ever been inducted into any Hall of Fame, based on honesty, their credibility or any other noble reason. Their qualifications are based solely on their ability to play the game and do the job they were hired to do. His admission must be determined on his ability to do the job he was hired to do and God will give him his rightful due.

God is even watching the State of Alabama and the way Judge Roy Moore was treated for following his instructions. Man has always wanted to be the Master rather than the Servant. Man seems to have forgotten that God has warned the world that 'he is a jealous God'. Judge Moore was right and complying with Divine instructions, even though he may believe that he was acting on his own. The Ten Commandments were the very first act of legislation of laws known to the civilized population in America. All of the existing laws in every State in the United States and every other Country are derivatives from the Ten Commandments. The Ten Commandments belongs in the Courthouse since the Courthouse is where the enforcement of these laws is conducted. The presence of the Ten Commandments in the Church is to teach us exactly what is allowed and permitted before these Commandments are violated and when they are violated, punishment is imposed in the Courthouse. God will touch the hearts of men in the Supreme Court to render a just decision on the issue involving the 'separation of Church and State'. There can be no separation because this Country was established and built on the concept religion is a vital part of our survival. God is deeply rooted in the moral fibers of America and in the hearts of men in decision-making positions. They are compelled to perform their duties for

69.

justice tempered with mercy and there can be no separation between Church and State. Even though this Country was established on the Christian faith, our Constitution allows the practice of other religions by others that immigrated in the United States from various foreign soils. Nevertheless, to allow immigrants to come into this Country and oppose our Christian traditions is like allowing a stranger to move into your home and change the rules you have for your home. They knew what your rules were before they came and if they have a problem with the house rules, then they should stay where they came from. No one should be allowed to change your house rules. They should be allowed to practice their religion, but not create changes to the American traditions. With respect to other religions, there must be a meeting of the minds as to the meaning or religious interpretation of the name or entity for 'GOD' since God is the essence of all religions being a 'Supreme Being', for recognition as a credible religion.

Even matters that relate to deceased individuals, God is aware of the wrongs that were inflicted upon them during their lifetime. The wrongful conduct of the National Football League refusing to induct Bob Hayes, No. 22 in the Hall of Fame because of his felony drug conviction is on the plans for God to touch that committee's members heart and give him everything he is entitled to have. Those members will recognize the fact the felony conviction had nothing to do with Mr. Hayes tenure as a member of the Dallas Cowboys and the N.F.L., and his accomplishments cannot be erased simply because of a single incident that involved an indiscretion act at the end of his career. God knows that Mr. Hayes earned that right and men with average intelligence has judged him in a manner that they would not want to be judged under similar circumstances. This is where forgiveness comes into play because that is the American way and he has served his Country well and with respect through his service in the Olympics. The world knows that other individuals have recorded faster time, but there has never been another track star the weighed from 180 to 200 pounds and ran that fast and there will never be another individual to do so within the next fifty years. No one can break his record unless they do so under the exact same circumstance the record was set and there has never been another athlete to do so.

Others runners merely set a record for their size and weight class but not the heavy weight class. That record will probably survive forever, as long as there is Track and Field events.

God also recognize the fact, the American Negro is the most hostile culture in America and is second only to Africans for destroying their own kind. The two cultures would rather help a member of other cultures than to help their own family members. My culture, the American Negro has copied from the Caucasian culture's methods to hide and conceal the past conduct of our ancestors. The very thing that the Caucasians despise is the exact same thing the Negro is proud of. Caucasians are constantly seeking ways to get their complexions darker and the Negroes are trying to get lighter complexions either through cosmetics or through mix cultures and some by marriage and union of the Caucasian and Negro cultures. Both cultures have a past history that they are ashamed of.

Caucasians keep religion out of the schools for fear their greatest fear will be discovered. Not realizing that the same fear is imposed upon 98% of the world and every one in the United States is likewise affected. It is the Caucasian blood mixed with African blood that created the Negro. Caucasian blood is mixed with every other culture, other than a few of the remaining tribes left in Africa. Every fear that the Caucasian has falls upon all other cultures at a slower rate. Those who have eyes and ears know exactly what is being said and it is not my place to elaborate any further. The Bible tells us to "seek and you shall find and ask and it shall be given unto you". Our problem is we don't ask and we try to find the answer on our own, which is impossible. We stumble and find views we want to be the truth on so many occasions and more frequently, fall short of the actual truth.

The Negro is ashamed of the humbleness and weakness of our ancestors that led to the slavery on the Negro culture. When God allows bad situations to arise he has a reason. The Negro culture has yet to see the good that came from slavery. The good that came from slavery on Negroes is the fact, not one single Negro has to get a "green card" as African's, and Mexican's and other foreign individuals have to get. The Caucasians are not the originators of slavery, it was the Africans and the curse that Noah placed on his grandson, Ham's son

75.

Canaan was the original form of slavery. The Negro is ashamed of the manner Negroes were introduced into the field of entertainment that the National Association for the Advancement of Colored People, (N.A.A.C.P.) had the federal courts to seal the Amos and Andy Shows from the public so they can never be seen again. The younger generation should be allowed to see what our ancestors had to do to get into the movies. This is a contamination of history and should not be allowed to stand. The banning of the Amos and Andy Show deprived their relatives of the opportunity to get the royalties from showing the movies in today's Entertainment market. The actions by the N.A.A.C.P. in sealing the rights to broadcast that show deprived Negroes that are the offspring of the characters that played the parts of their rightful inheritance. It is this type of conduct that hurts the Negro. The American Negro is the most confusing culture of all and there is no way Negroes can learn to understand each other but other cultures are constantly trying to find ways to appease the mass of the affluent Negroes. The Negro culture by its very nature is a contradicting culture. During the days of segregation, the demands by the Negro as applied to maintain segregation in balance was to have separate but equal facilities if integration between the Caucasians and Negroes could not be accepted. When integration of the two cultures became a reality, the Negro educational institutions wanted to cling to traditional Black Historical status to preserve the Negro culture, not realizing that is the exact same reason why segregation of the cultures

77.

existed. The late George Wallace, Governor for Alabama stood in the doorway at the University of Alabama in an attempt to keep Negro students from attending, in an attempt to preserve the Historical White status. Caucasian and Negro educational institutions eventually integrated. Integration allowed mixed cultures to attend colleges as students. Negroes wanted to be allowed to work and hold any position at traditionally White educational institutions that is allowed to Caucasians, but are not willing to allow Caucasians to hold high positions at Historical Black Colleges as presidents. The Black Caucus in the United States Congress and various state's refuses to allow Caucasians to join and serve with them as a member of the caucus. The Negroes wanted to be able to compete in the Miss America Beauty Pageant and eventually Vanessa Williams was allowed to be a contestant. She won and the officials found a way to take her crown away. The Negroes created their own Miss Black America Beauty Pageant and they refuse to allow Caucasians to compete as contestants. The creation of the 'Affirmative Action Program' was designed to make it possible for Negroes to compete and to enter into the corporate world because minorities have been systematically excluded and discriminated against and denied this opportunity. This program was not available to members of the Caucasian culture, even though there are members of the Caucasian culture that are denied the equal opportunity to enter into the corporate segment. To appease that certain segment of the Negro culture many Caucasians were laid off and some dismissed from employment to make room to hire Negroes since they had been systematically discriminated against and could not get into the mainstream of employment. Negroes were not concerned about the reverse discrimination being imposed upon Caucasians. In fact, those who benefited from the 'Affirmative Action Program' were not even concerned because that program did not apply to all Negroes, as long as they had a steak on their table each day, the house of their dream and a car of their choice. This is the selfish attitude that has held the Negro culture down. The Negroes that are blessed with the opportunities to succeed treat other Negroes worst that the members of the Caucasian culture. Even in private employment when the Negro's own their own business. They use the exact same discriminating policies to refuse

80.

to hire other Negroes that are less fortunate than they are. Many Negroes and Caucasians that lived on the poverty level are treated exactly the same and most of them having experienced a hard luck streak in their life at some point, had to experience a criminal prosecution in order to provide for their families. The creation of the background system showing a criminal conviction keeps them from being hired on many occasions. Those having the power to hire these people and give them a chance to provide for their families, fail to realize that their own parents in most cases were convicted felons because of acts of indiscretion to provide support for them. If a reasonable guess had to be made, I would say about 70% of Negroes over the age of forty (40) years and 60% of Caucasians over the age of forty (40) have some kind of criminal prosecution on their record. Many as far back as twenty to thirty years and employers refuse to hire these people because of a single infraction. Many sincere individuals are forced back into a life of crime to survive because they do not have the mental skills to maneuver around that obstacle. The problem with this process, Negroes and poor Caucasians learned how to make illegal money, but lacked the education and skills to know how to keep their money and property. Caucasians and the Negroes that had a chance to get an education learned how to take the money and property from the poor segment that managed to acquire a portion of success to have money and property, as public servants. It seems as though the various forms of government is designed to prevent poor people of all culture from being

83.

successful. Since the criminal justice process is a booming business, it appears that the government on all levels would rather have the jails and prisons filled to maximum capacity rather than allow poor people to be successful. God is aware of all that has been discussed, as well as the fact various courts are filled with individuals, serving as judges, that many are incapable of rendering decisions in the interest of justice and tempered with mercy. Negroes are being subjected to life sentence without the possibility of a parole at a record high of seven to one for the exact same crimes that are being committed by Caucasians. Judges are subjecting defendants on parole and probation to random drug test that they can't even pass. Every act where abuse of discretion is involved, God will subject a punishment on

84.

those closest to those in power so it will manifest the contempt that God has for such actions. When arrogance prevent them from complying with the sworn duty for the positions they hold, God will remove them from such positions of authority. It is this kind of conduct that compels God to act out of anger without hesitation or reservation and mercy is shown in accord with that as shown by them on others. They refuse to render justice toward others, as they would have imposed upon them, if they were in the same or similar positions and under the same circumstances. They took those positions with a clear understanding "to judge not that ye be not judged", and they choose to be disobedient and do as they please. God has always reacted for disobedience but those in power being without eyes to see and without ears to hear have not noticed God's retribution out of arrogance. The only thing they realize that they are sick from an illness due to hard luck or a bad streak of luck at a time they believed to be at the peak of their success. These individuals have a strong respect for medical doctors and they fail to realize that not one single one of them has ever been cured through medical treatment. Life was simply prolonged, but not cured. It is your own decisions that determine your future.

Chapter 4

God's Instructions for Cure

Man has always tried to protect his health by selecting the proper diet. In spite of the fact, God has previously instructed man that, "It is not what goes into the mouth that defiles the body, but that which comes out of the body". [Paraphrasing]

Since it is clear that the food we eat cannot harm the body, according to the word. Let's discuss that which can defile the body and cause sickness to plague our body. Accordingly, we must get a clear understanding that only words can come out of the mouth that can defile the body:

1.One of the reasons is, we have been instructed 'not to bear false witness against our neighbors.' When someone tell you something that they saw, it may be the truth when they told you. However, when you repeat what they told you, it is no longer the truth because you can only testify to that you have actually seen and heard for yourself. When you repeat something that was told to you, you are bearing false witness against your neighbor if you did not actually see or hear what you are repeating. In fact, you do not even know if that was the truth that was told to you. That is one act that initiated a phase of defiling your body.

2. When we get angry words are said that cannot be taken back. Even though you may apologize, the words were said and a seed was planted in the mind of the person you are talking to. Remember in previous Chapters we learned that words have power and can hurt someone.

3. When these words are spoken, another process has further defiled the body. Even though God made man in his image, there is no evident that he had a sense of humor as man does. Accordingly this must be attributed through man's ability to exercise 'free will' to amuse himself. Even though words are used in a joking manner the words still have the same power as though they are being said in a serious manner. The wrong words used in a joking manner can create further actions to defile the body.

4. You may have the view that you have not said anything that could be considered harmful to defile the body. Probably not, but one or many of your ancestors may have. Remember when Noah caused a curse to fall upon his grandson for the actions of Ham, you can also

be carrying the burden for one or more of your ancestors. When this process go for years without going through the process of lightening the load of these sins, they increase and cause an unbearable load on the soul, which cause a reaction that defiles the body through various kind of sickness. To give a clear understanding of the process that is discussed above, you can probably relate to the occasions when your body reaches its maximum capacity for food, you get an uncomfortable feeling and immediately you know that you need a laxative to get relief from constipation. Your soul function in exactly the same manner. It is the forgiveness for your sins that provide the relief of unloading these sins. In St. Matthew 18:21 Peter asked Jesus how many times must he forgive his brother for sins against him. Jesus replied in St.

Matthew 18:22, that he should forgive him seventy times seven a day. In essence, there is no limitation of times to forgive another for the transgressions against you. You should be willing to forgive a person as many times as you would want to be forgiven for you're sin against him. The Catholic Church use the process of confession to a Priest to comply with the fact that when two or more gather in the name of the Father, he is also present. However, I am led to say that "but, except ye repent, ye shall all likewise perish" [St. Luke 13:3] and however many people that you sin before is the exact or greater amount that you must repent before, which direct you to the Church. You must say specifically what it is you want to be forgiven for, exactly as you would say to a priest. It does not necessarily have to be the Church, but people that can hear and understand what you are saying and even family and friends can be included. To repent, you do not have to name the person your transgression was directed towards, but you have to say what you did to deserve being forgiven for. This is the key to starting the healing process. God knows that men in positions of authority will act through arrogance and refuse to do what is required and would rather be damned and lose their souls out of pride before asking for forgiveness. Pride is the vanity of a foolish person. To repent, God is not interested in the name of persons the sin was committed against because he already knows that. He knows that men in positions of authority will be required to make decisions that will injure a few for the good of the mass. Nevertheless, a sin was committed. He has an understanding heart, but you must ask for forgiveness. Unless you repent and specifically ask for forgiveness, the prescription medications are nothing more than placing a bandage over a cancer. When the medication does not heal the sickness, or the recovery process appears to show no improvement, your sins are too great for the small forgiveness that you requested. Go back to the source and repent for matters that you have forgotten, or those that may have been committed by your ancestors. Certainly you cannot name their wrongful deeds, so ask for forgiveness for the burdens that you are carrying that was caused by your ancestors. Repeat this process on a daily basis, as frequent as you can until you can see an improvement. Even if a recovery is not obtain, the soul is relieved from the sins and peace will be achieved. Remember, it is not the recovery from the sickness that you are seeking, the main objective is to save your soul. Sometimes recovery is the reward when you act with a sincere heart and ask for forgiveness. To repent merely set the healing process in motion to respond with the proper medication. Doctors have recognized the fact prayer has aided speedy recovery in-patients and on some occasions the recovery even amazed the doctors. You are not to misunderstand the message in this book. God has given man the intelligence to create ways to recover from illness through medicine. There are many occasions when the medication do not work, but when the sins are light on the soul, the healing process can began. There is no way you can began to estimate how much prayer is necessary, or the number of sins that has defiled your body and don't even try to guess. Make it a constant ritual to pray all through the day and ask for forgiveness for all of the sins that you can name individually and can remember. For sins that you cannot remember, add to the prayer by asking for forgiveness of the sins that has escaped your memory and that you are asking for forgiveness with a sincere and humble heart. Be mindful that God takes pleasure in knowing that you have placed your life and future in his hands.

God is aware of the fact some of his creations refuse to acknowledge and recognize him as being the 'Supreme Being'. There are individuals that made statements that they did not believe in God, but little that they knew at the time, they did believe in God. Every lip that has ever uttered the word "GOD" had knowledge of his existence and having that knowledge imbedded the belief of the existence of God in their minds and hearts. They were probably disgruntled because their prayers were not answered when they wanted them the most, or for allowing something to happen in their lives that made them unhappy. At any rate, the knowledge of God is evident that they believed in the existence of God. Even though Satan worshipers chose a deity of their own, fail to realize that even Satan believe in God. In fact, he believed in God so much that he wanted to be God and control the heavens while he was Lucifer. God being a just and jealous God, he gave Lucifer an alternative kingdom and a new name that he has to this day. If Satan believe in God, certainly his follower's has the knowledge and believes in God as the 'Supreme Being'. Again just because individuals say the do not believe in God, do not necessarily mean that. If they have the knowledge of God, then they also believe in God. The lack of knowledge on the existence of God is the only way an individual cannot believe in God. No one can believe in anything that they have no knowledge of.

Chapter 5

God's Revelation

In the next four years God will direct more attention to individuals that travels under the cloak of religion with less than sincere intentions, as well as those who takes an oath on the Bible without being sincere with the obligations that accompanies the oath that is taken. He will expose the truth to the public about issues that are desired and meant to be kept as secrets. We all know that God has knowledge about all secrets that exist. He will touch the hearts of the few that will gain information and lead them to the proper sources to expose them for what they are. He will have no compassion or mercy for those that acted in a complete disregard for feelings of others that resulted in shame and embarrassment without a just cause. He will avenge the innocent for the suffering that they endured unjustly and the world will see it all happen and wonder why such drastic measures can be imposed upon one individual. The punishment inflicted will be in proportion to the harm that they caused upon others measured over a thousand times. Be wise and not share sympathy because you being the readers have no clue as to what that individual has done to cause such a drastic punishment. An act of compassion and sympathy can invite that punishment towards you. These incidents will rise to the surface so often the world will take notice on a mass scale. Even the unknown individuals will attract world wide news coverage and every act of conspiracy will be brought to the surface for exposure.

Men in the most powerful positions, not only in the United States, but world wide and all religions proclaim to have faith in God, but God will reveal the fact their faith is in worldly values and not in him. Their actions are as a man with a bottomless well full of water, but store hundreds of gallons of water in their possession, in case the well run dry. They do not have enough faith to believe that God will provide a lifetime supply of water, regardless of the water situation on earth. This is the concept that is used by individuals that value monetary values over human life. God takes pride in providing for those that tries to love one another as he has loved us. No one has ever completely done so because our selfish attitudes and desires for great security and comfort will not permit us to completely let go. We are all within that

100.

category, no matter what we say, or how hard we try, there is no evident that a single person anywhere have successfully done so, in obedience with God's instructions to love one another as he have loved us. He knows that when he allowed 'free will' to influence our lives, man will always find reasons to justify the inability to love one another. Man has convinced himself that one culture is superior to another, but in reality, no culture is superior to the other and there was only one color of man in the beginning and there is only one color of man today. We just happened to be of different complexions that resulted from a Divine engineering project that God allowed. None of us had anything to do with that project and we must realize that when our parents discipline one of our siblings, we love them just the same.

101.

Chapter Six

Developing a Relationship with your Angel

I am led to discuss my understanding of Angels as they relate to every individual. Even though there are ancient and well known angels that has been around since their creation, new angels are created with each individual. They serve as guides and protectors to direct each individual on their chosen path. Not every individual gets the opportunity to follow their chosen path. Many individuals through the exercise of 'free will' fail to listen to their guardian angel and take a path of their own. When they realize their presence is unappreciated, they leave and return periodical to see if there are changes that require them to stay with the individual. Sometimes there are changes and on so many occasions many individuals go through life stumbling without any since of guidance and refuse to listen to anyone. Like everything else, there are exceptions to every rule. A prudent person will understand at the early stages of life when they need help. They will seek guidance and pray for guidance. These prayers even though directed to God immediately alerts that angel to return on duty.

Angels are sensitive and have the exact same qualities as man. They have emotions as well and will abandon their assigned post if their presence is not appreciated. The greatest problem with man, he fails to establish a relationship with the assigned angel because no one has ever told them they had an angel, or how to establish a relationship with the angel.

At some point in your life an idea came to you, or your mind told you to do a specific thing, in a complete surprise. This is your angel trying to give you guidance. The very first thought that you get is the angel, but you must also realize that you also have a dark angel that will try to lead you in the wrong direction and it takes pleasure in seeing you suffer. The doubt that comes after you get the first impression is the dark angel trying to lead you away from your blessing. Surprisingly as it may seem, most people follow the dark angel and miss their blessings. Always expel any notion of doubt from your mind and always act with confidence and follow your first impression.

You should be aware of the fact all angels do not like each other. You may have a friend and your angel do not particular care for your friend's angel. If you share your thoughts and blessings with your friend, your angel in all probability, stop giving you blessings. Your angel knows something about your friend that you may not know. Your friend may not mean you good as you may believe and want you to be unsuccessful. Angels know when people want to be your friend as long as you do not be more successful than they are. Angles will tolerate that friendship as long as you do not share the thoughts and blessings in store for you. It is an old ancient belief that people can steal your blessings by asking you for something of value before 12:00 Noon. Many times they will have money, but will ask you for $1.00 and when you pass that bill or coins, you are also passing you luck and blessings. If you must lend money, lay it down on

105.

some kind of surface and let them pick it up. By doing this, you are not passing your blessings.

You may get a sudden urge to play a specific number in a lottery. This is your angel trying to communicate with you. That angel knows your needs and desires and will try to help you. These sudden urges you keep to yourself. You can share your success but not your blessings and luck. That angel's feelings are exactly like yours. When you are on your job, you don't want someone else or another business to profit from your labor, unless they are paying you too. This is the same concept angels have. Any visions that you may get, keep it to yourself and you will get these kind of blessing more frequent and more abundantly. The more you listen to your angel, the more they will try to make you happy.

They take pride in doing their job well. When you are happy, they are happy also. It is important that you listen to the very first thoughts that come to you. That is your connection with your angel. Never share that thought with anyone. Communications between you and your angel are privilege and not meant to be shared. Guidance between you and your angel is as close as you can get to divine guidance. If you listen, your angel will guide you to a level of success you could not believe possible. Sit in a quite location whenever you can with your eyes close. Try to make your mind blank by not thinking about anything. Concentrate on a blank. This is the only path an angel can travel. Whatever comes to your mind during this process will be your guidance. Create a diet that consists of mostly sea foods, poultry and vegetables.

www.ingramcontent.com/pod-product-compliance
Lightning Source LLC
Chambersburg PA
CBHW050538280326
41933CB00011B/1630